STRETCH! RELAX! ENERGIZE! FOR HIKERS, BIKERS & PADDLERS

ERIN WIDMAN

PHOTOGRAPHS BY DONNA DAY

SASQUATCH BOOKS
SEATTLE

Published by Sasquatch Books, Seattle
Printed in Hong Kong
Distributed in Canada by Raincoast Books, Ltd.
03 02 01 00 99   5 4 3 2 1

Cover and interior design: Kate Basart
Yoga postures photographs: Copyright ©1999 by Donna Day

Library of Congress Cataloging in Publication Data
Widman, Erin. 1970–
        Sleeping bag yoga / Erin Widman : photographs by Donna Day.
              p. cm.
        ISBN 1-57061-165-3
        1. Yoga—Popular works. 2. Outdoor life—Health aspects. I. Title.
        RA781.7.W536 1999
        613.7'046—dc21   98-41007

SASQUATCH BOOKS / 615 Second Avenue / Seattle, Washington 98104 / (206)467-4300
www.SasquatchBooks.com/books@SasquatchBooks.com

Sasquatch Books publishes high-quality adult nonfiction and children's books related to the Northwest (Alaska to San Francisco). For more information about Sasquatch Books titles, contact us at the address above, or view our site on the World Wide Web.

► contents

► introduction

I was two months into the excursion of a lifetime: bicycle touring, backpacking, and kayaking in New Zealand and Asia. Having just completed a leg of high-mountain trekking, I was returning to my main mode of transportation, cycling. I was in the best physical and mental shape of my life, yet the prospect of pedaling up mountainous roads seemed daunting. A chronic tightness in my neck was leaving my spirits dragging. Unless something changed, I didn't see how I could complete my travels—let alone enjoy myself.

During one of those inevitable moments of longing for the comforts of home, I realized what was missing. I was pushing my capabilities to the limit on this demanding trip without paying any attention to my body's subtle needs. Back in Seattle I was typically on my yoga mat every day, tending to my physical and mental well-being. On this trip, I hadn't practiced yoga once. With all the new places to explore and the challenges of pedaling, hiking, and paddling, I simply had not given myself time.

One morning, as I was considering easing my stiff body out of the tent, it occurred to me that my sleeping pad and bag were roughly the same size as my yoga mat back home, and that they could serve the same purpose. Turning over in my sleeping bag, I pushed up into a position called "downward facing dog." Replaying the quiet voice of my yoga instructor while stretching my back was exactly what I needed.

During the rest of my trip, I developed a series of yoga positions that could be executed in a limited space—inside my small backpacking tent, either in or on top of my sleeping bag. From the broad array of yoga positions, I was able to select those that stretched, relaxed, and energized the specific muscles that had tightened during a strenuous day of hiking, cycling, or paddling. Soon, the tightness in my neck disappeared and I succeeded in reaching my destinations with body relaxed and spirit soaring.

You don't have to be an extreme-sports activist to derive benefits from *Sleeping Bag Yoga*, nor do you need any previous yoga experience. These routines have been culled from an ancient system of body work, with simplicity and safety in mind. If you kayak and beach camp for a few days, your upper body will get a workout as your lower body stiffens in the tight compartment of your boat. Stretching at the end of the day will be soothing and relaxing. A routine in the morning will revitalize you for another day of paddling. Yoga can confer similar benefits when you're hiking—whether it's months on the Pacific Crest Trail or an overnight in the Olympic Mountains. Yoga enhances the body's capabilities, and the positions in this book enhance the abilities of paddlers, hikers, and cyclists.

1 twiLight position

1 Sit on or between heels, with knees parted slightly, hips facing squarely forward, and weight distributed equally on both sitbones.

2 With hands resting lightly on thighs, extend spine upward.

3 Inhale and exhale slowly, expanding lungs and rib cage in all directions as you breathe into every cell.

yoga tip Place a folded-up sleeping bag under your sitbones to provide support.

► HOW to use sLeeping Bag yoga

This book describes and illustrates twenty yoga positions organized in a sequence to reach all major muscle groups while requiring minimal body movement as you progress from one position to the next—certainly an asset when you are performing these routines inside a tent. I have done all of the positions in *Sleeping Bag Yoga* while inside my mummy-style sleeping bag. Although it requires some twisting and scrunching, it's possible. But these positions can be executed just as well on top of your sleeping bag, inside or outside your tent.

These icons identify specific positions as being especially beneficial to hikers 🚶 paddlers 🛶 or cyclists 🚴. The accompanying photographs show the final positions to work toward.

Ending a day of vigorous exercise by executing the positions in the order they appear in the book will take your body to a relaxed state. In the morning, start from the back of the book and work your way forward to energize yourself. The most important guideline, however, is to do what your body and spirit are asking for; I believe our bodies know instinctively what's right for us. Feel free to pick and choose the positions that seem right for a given day.

At the end of the book is a separate group of positions, called the Strengthening Series. These exercises require more space than is available in a tent and more consciousness of your body's limitations. Building strength and endurance is easier and more effective when the body is in proper alignment (any cyclist who has ridden an ill-fitting bike knows the cost of misalignment—ouch!). The series emphasizes proper body alignment as a key to strengthening the torso (the back and chest muscles), for when your torso is strong, you have more endurance. In a kayak, for example, the arms may hold the paddle, but it's the torso that does much of the work. Similarly, a hiker with a 30-pound backpack feels the exhaustion in the torso before the legs give out.

Here are some basic guidelines to help you develop your *Sleeping Bag Yoga* practice:

- Move slowly. Don't rush to try to achieve the final position.
- Use your exhaled breaths to move deeper into a position, releasing slightly on your inhaled breaths.
- Stay in each position for at least 10 slow breaths.
- Engage only the specific muscles needed to maintain the position, releasing all others.
- As you breathe, focus your attention on the specific muscles you have used throughout the day.
- Keep your facial muscles relaxed and soft.
- Close your eyes or maintain a soft gaze.
- Move slowly and mindfully between positions.

There is nothing quite as exhilarating as traveling under your own power across a beautiful landscape. Practicing *Sleeping Bag Yoga* can enhance your body's health, balance, and strength, so that you can fully enjoy each mountain pass, coastal strip, and country road.

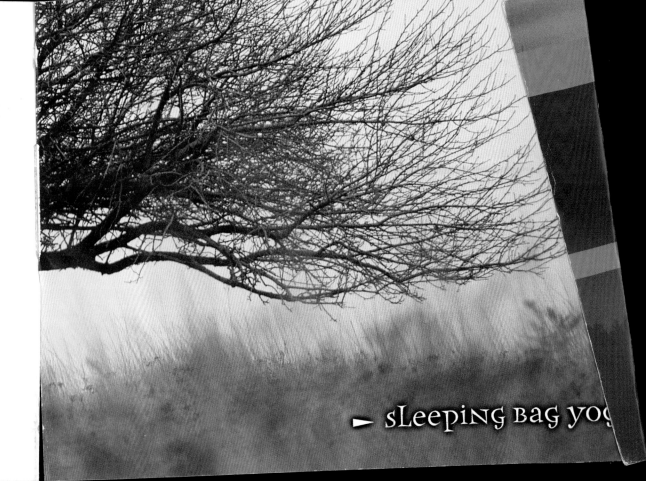

- sLeepiNG BaG yog

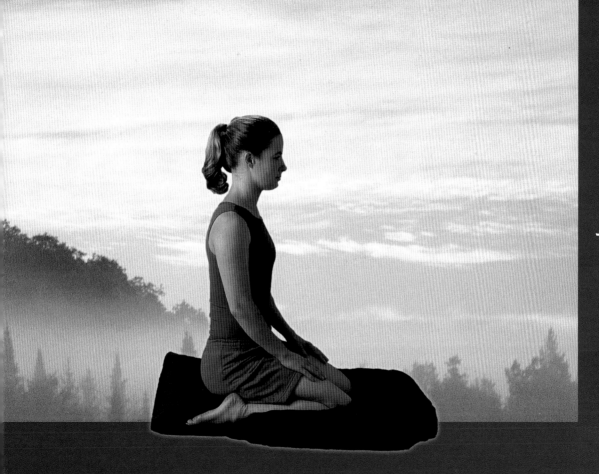

2 moonlight position

1 From Twilight Position, bow head forward, keeping spine extended.

2 Draw shoulder blades downward.

3 Release neck muscles, allowing gravity to take the weight of your head.

yoga tip Continue supporting yourself with a folded-up sleeping bag placed under your sitbones.

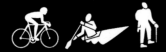

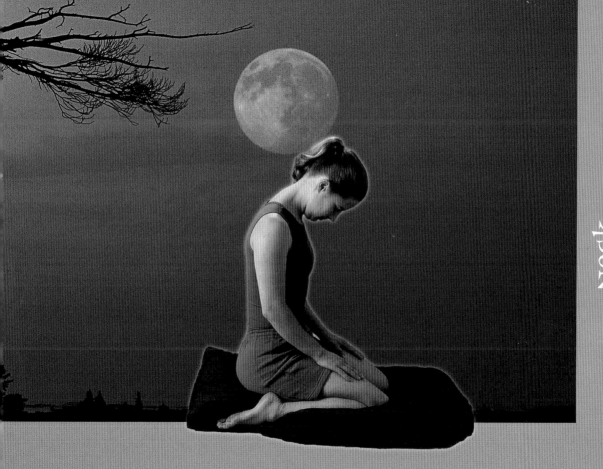

neck

3 ocean swell position

1 From Moonlight Position, shift forward, placing palms on ground directly beneath shoulders, with knees directly under hips.

2 Exhale slowly and smoothly, lifting mid-spine and belly upward while dropping head, pushing ground away with arms, and drawing shoulder blades away from each other.

3 Inhale slowly and smoothly, dropping mid-spine and belly downward while curving head, chest, and sitbones upward and pulling shoulder blades together.

4 As you exhale and inhale, feel each breath travel the entire length of your spine.

sLeepiNg Bag tip Using a large stuff sack with compression straps makes packing easier and keeps the carrying size small.

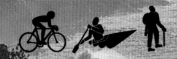

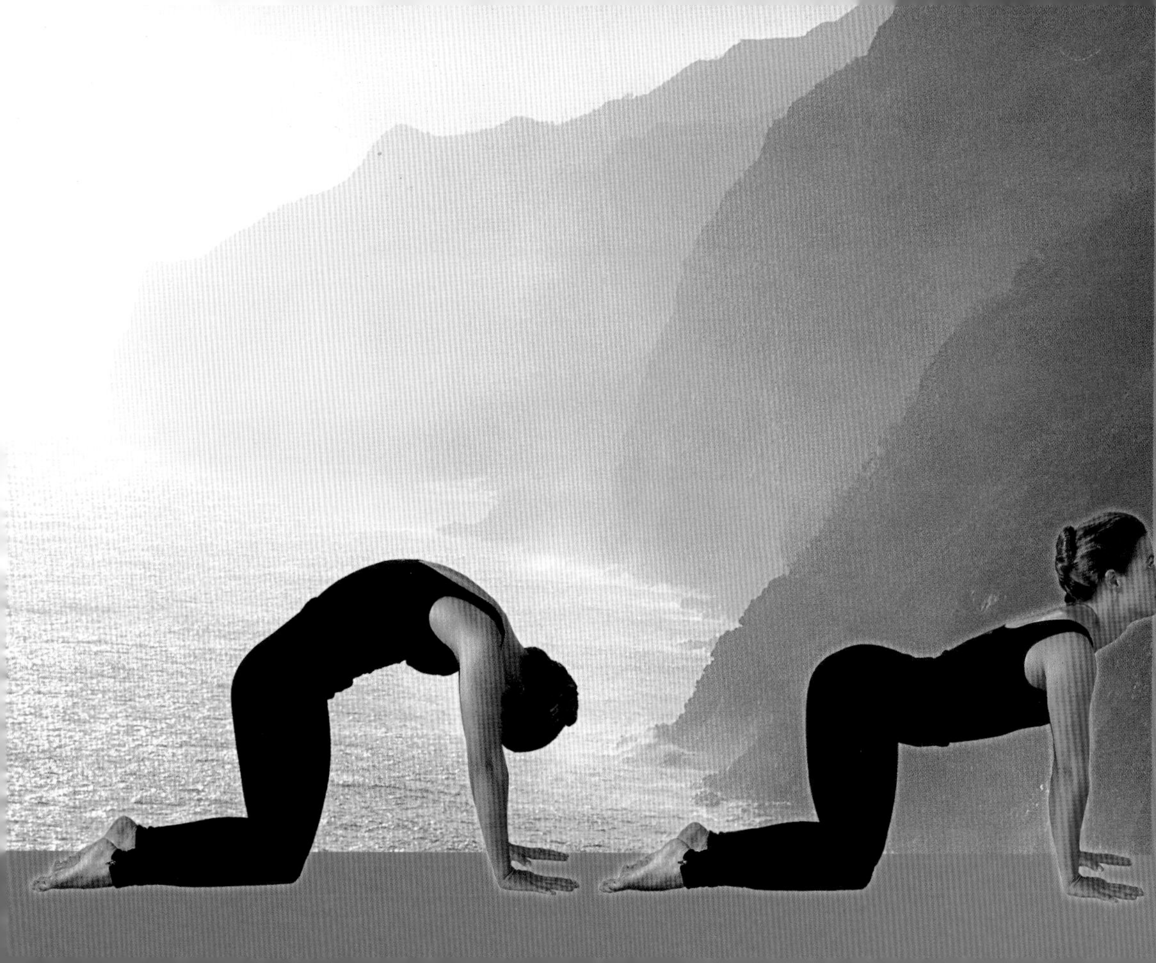

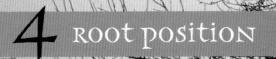

4 root position

1 From Ocean Swell Position, tuck toes under, placing balls of feet on ground.

2 Sink hips down toward heels, resting weight on heels to stretch the soles of your feet.

3 With head down, reach arms forward as if to slide fingertips under the earth.

yoga tip Push part of your sleeping bag against the back of your knees, under your thighs, to help alleviate any knee pain.

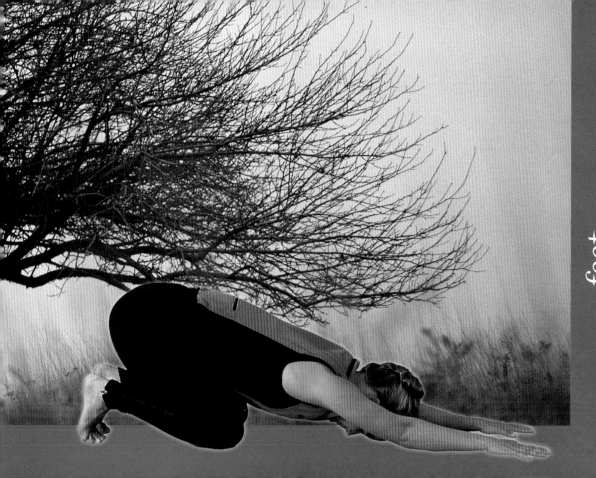

5 mountain pass position

1 From Root Position, straighten legs, moving pelvis squarely up and back while keeping feet and knees parallel and head down.

2 Stretch up and out of your wrists, elbows, and shoulders while dropping chest toward ground.

3 Inhale and exhale slowly, allowing the traction you've created to lengthen your spine.

yoga tip You can practice most *Sleeping Bag Yoga* positions inside your sleeping bag, to keep yourself warm.

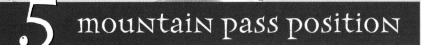

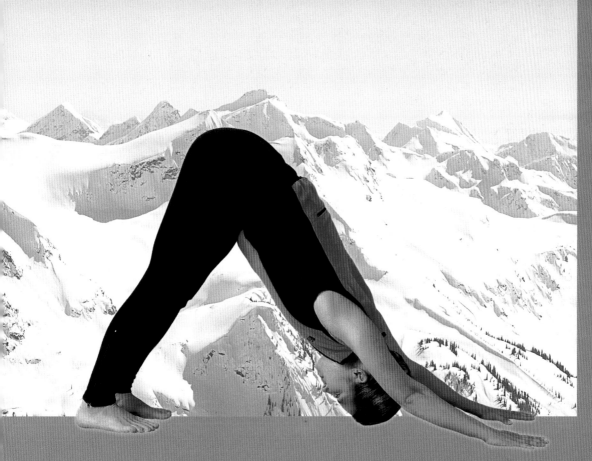

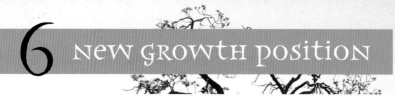

6 NEW GROWTH POSITION

1 From Mountain Pass Position, round spine forward until shoulder blades are over hands. Keeping lower back long, drop pelvis and press chest forward.

2 Stretch upward with the crown of head and outward with the bottoms of heels.

3 Use the strength in your quadriceps to propel more height into the front of your body.

sLeepiNg Bag tip Using a plastic bag inside of the stuff sack keeps the bag dry during any weather conditions and protects the plastic from tearing.

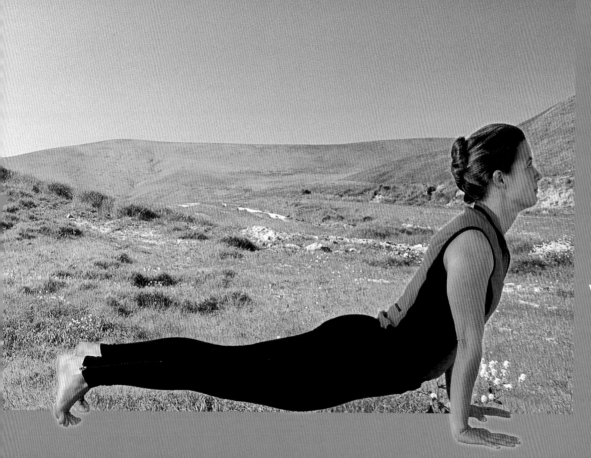

7 head wind position

1 From New Growth Position, bring one foot forward to between hands, bending knee under chest.

2 Stretch thighs strongly away from each other, keeping chest facing forward.

3 Let pelvis sink squarely downward, allowing the front leg's strength and structure to hold you.

4 Repeat with opposite side.

sleeping bag tip Placing your sleeping bag on top of the back rack while cycle touring allows more room in the panniers without affecting wind resistance.

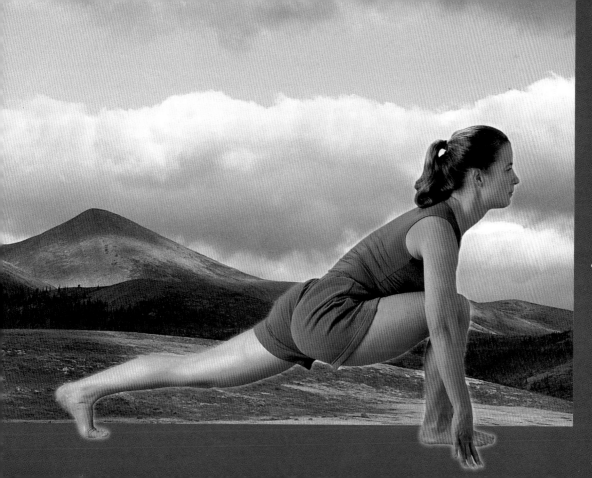

8 whirlpool position

1. Sit with weight balanced evenly on both sitbones. Bend left knee, placing foot solidly on the ground as if to stand. Curl right hand around bent knee and place left hand on ground behind pelvis for support.

2. Lengthening torso upward while tilting upper pelvis forward, rotate belly and upper torso toward bent knee, using the hand on the bent knee for leverage.

3. Spiral each vertebra as far around its axis as your breath allows.

4. Repeat on opposite side.

yoga tip   Sit on a folded-up sleeping bag to help tilt your pelvis forward.

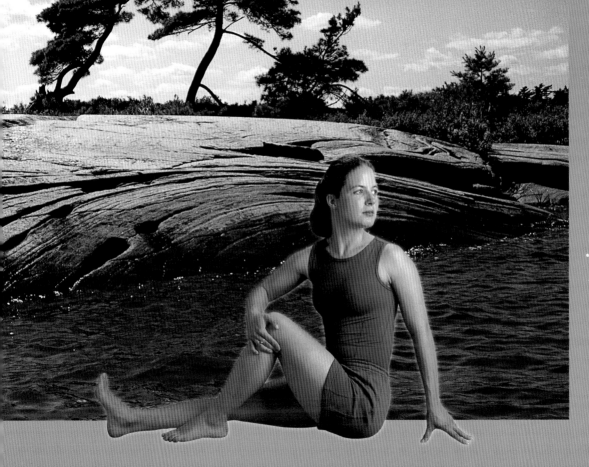

spine

9 sunrise position

1 From Whirlpool Position, extend right leg out at an angle and bend left foot into groin. Place right hand or elbow on inside of straightened knee.

2 Reach left arm up and over your ear, lengthening side waist parallel along straightened leg.

3 Twist torso upward and left shoulder back. Use each exhalation to move deeper into the twist.

4 Repeat with opposite side.

sleeping bag tip Placing the sleeping bag up high in the front compartment of your kayak keeps the bow light, easing your glide through the water.

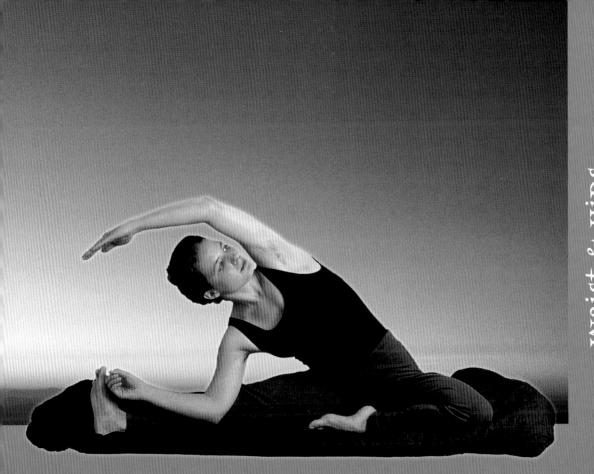

10 ◈ sunset position

1 From Sunrise Position, rotate front torso downward over straightened leg, bringing chest to face knee.

2 Tilt upper pelvis forward, releasing belly toward knee.

3 Holding onto leg for support, lower chest toward straightened leg by pulling thigh bone deep into pelvis.

4 Repeat with opposite side.

yoga tip Bunch a sleeping bag on top of your leg to rest your head on, or under your knee to release your hamstrings.

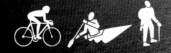

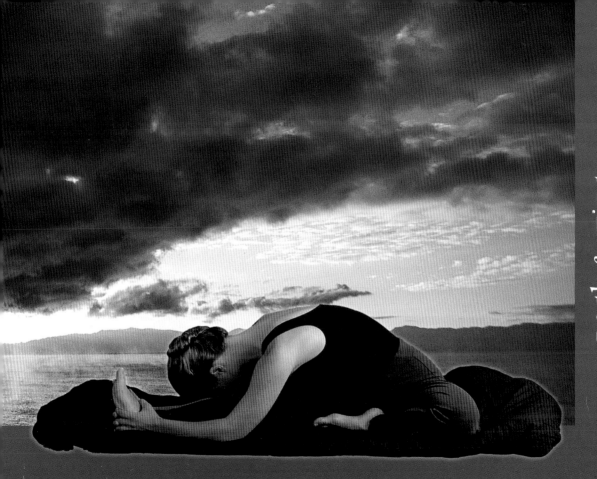

11 RIVER ROCK POSITION

1 From Sunset Position, straighten both legs out in front of you, balancing weight evenly on sitbones.

2 Extend belly up and over legs, lengthening entire spine.

3 Feel the motion of your breathing flow up and over your knees by releasing your hamstrings slightly as you inhale and deepening the stretch as you exhale.

yoga tip Bunch your sleeping bag under slightly bent knees to help release your lower back.

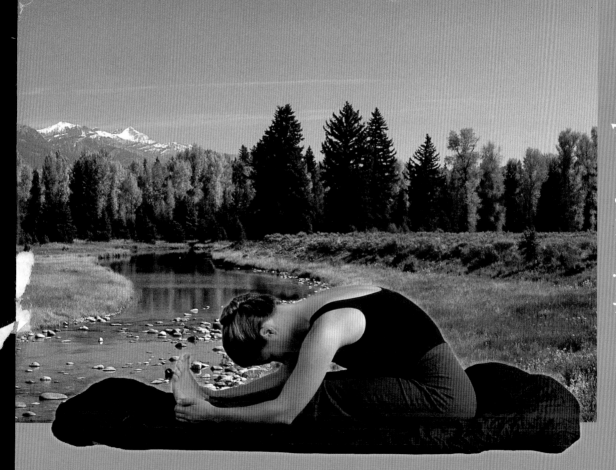

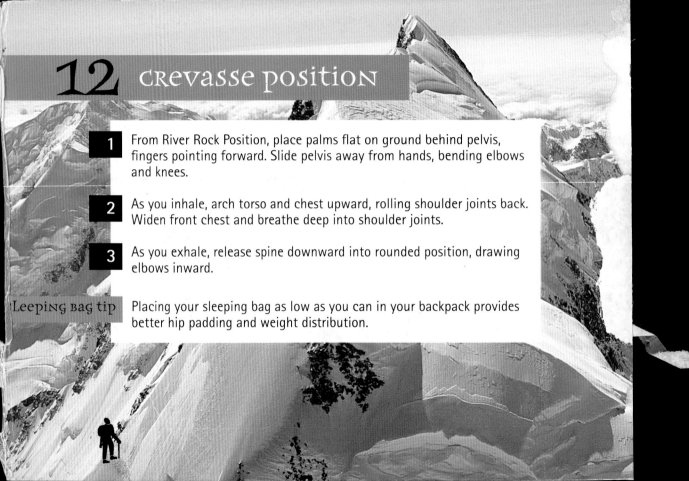

12 crevasse position

1 From River Rock Position, place palms flat on ground behind pelvis, fingers pointing forward. Slide pelvis away from hands, bending elbows and knees.

2 As you inhale, arch torso and chest upward, rolling shoulder joints back. Widen front chest and breathe deep into shoulder joints.

3 As you exhale, release spine downward into rounded position, drawing elbows inward.

Leeping bag tip Placing your sleeping bag as low as you can in your backpack provides better hip padding and weight distribution.

Shoulders & Chest

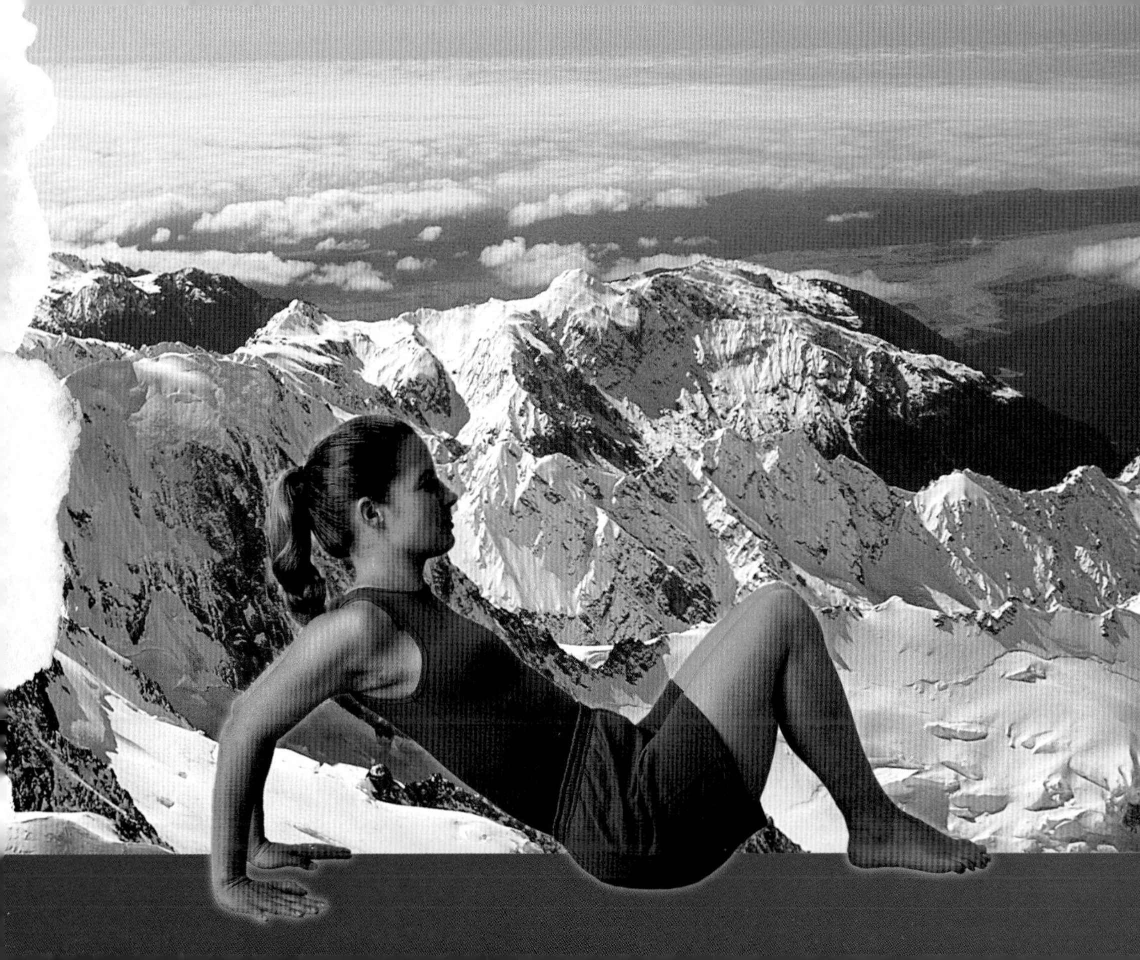

13 arches position

1 From Crevasse Position, lie back, keeping feet hip width apart. Leaving head and shoulders on ground, lift chest and pelvis upward. Engage quadriceps strongly to create a right angle with knees.

2 Interlock fingers on ground under pelvis. Press upper arms downward, rolling shoulders open and back.

3 Lift spine deep into body, supporting yourself with shoulders and feet.

yoga tip Place an evenly folded sleeping bag under your shoulders to lessen the pressure on your neck.

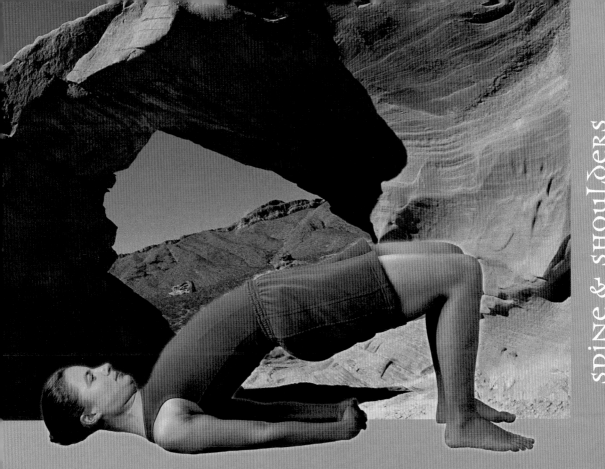

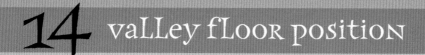

14 vaLLey fLoor position

1 From Arches Position, rest entire length of spine on ground. Place soles of feet together, bending knees out to the sides and relaxing shoulders and arms.

2 Lengthen lower back by tilting pubic bone upward, keeping whole spine on ground.

3 Allow gravity to take hold of legs, releasing tension in inner thighs.

yoga tip Bunch up a sleeping bag under your knees for support.

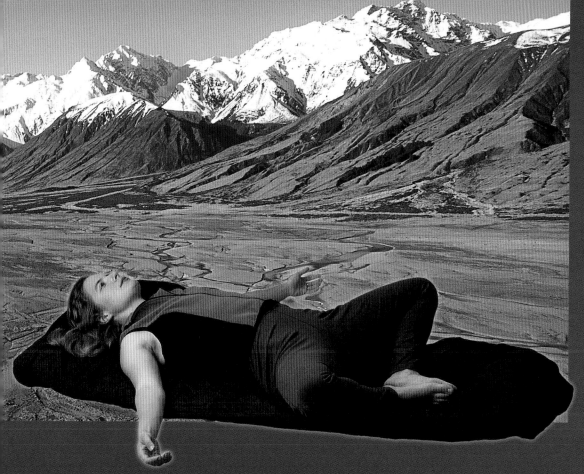

inner thighs

15 nurse Log position

1 From Valley Floor Position, pull knees in toward shoulders and hold feet directly above knees.

2 Breathe deeply as you pull feet and legs downward, lengthening lower spine.

sleeping bag tip Putting your socks and other clothing in the sleeping bag overnight will warm them for dressing on chilly mornings.

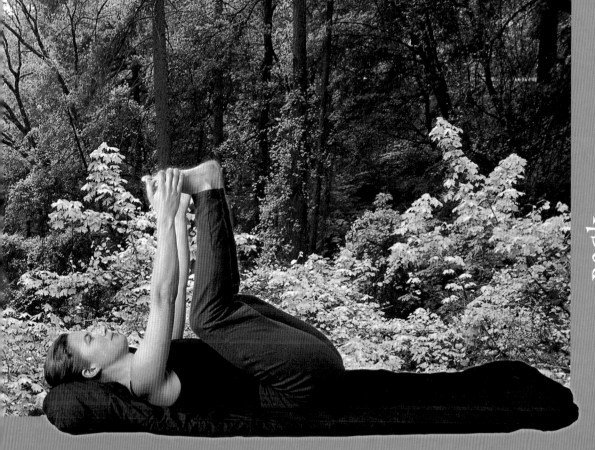

16 switchback position

1 From Nurse Log Position, release right leg and place left foot on right knee. Wrap hands around back of right thigh.

2 Holding back of thigh, push angled left knee away from body while using right knee to draw left foot toward chest.

3 With your breathing, focus on the deep muscles in your buttocks.

4 Repeat with opposite side.

yoga tip Lay sleeping bag out flat beneath you to ensure that your spine is in alignment.

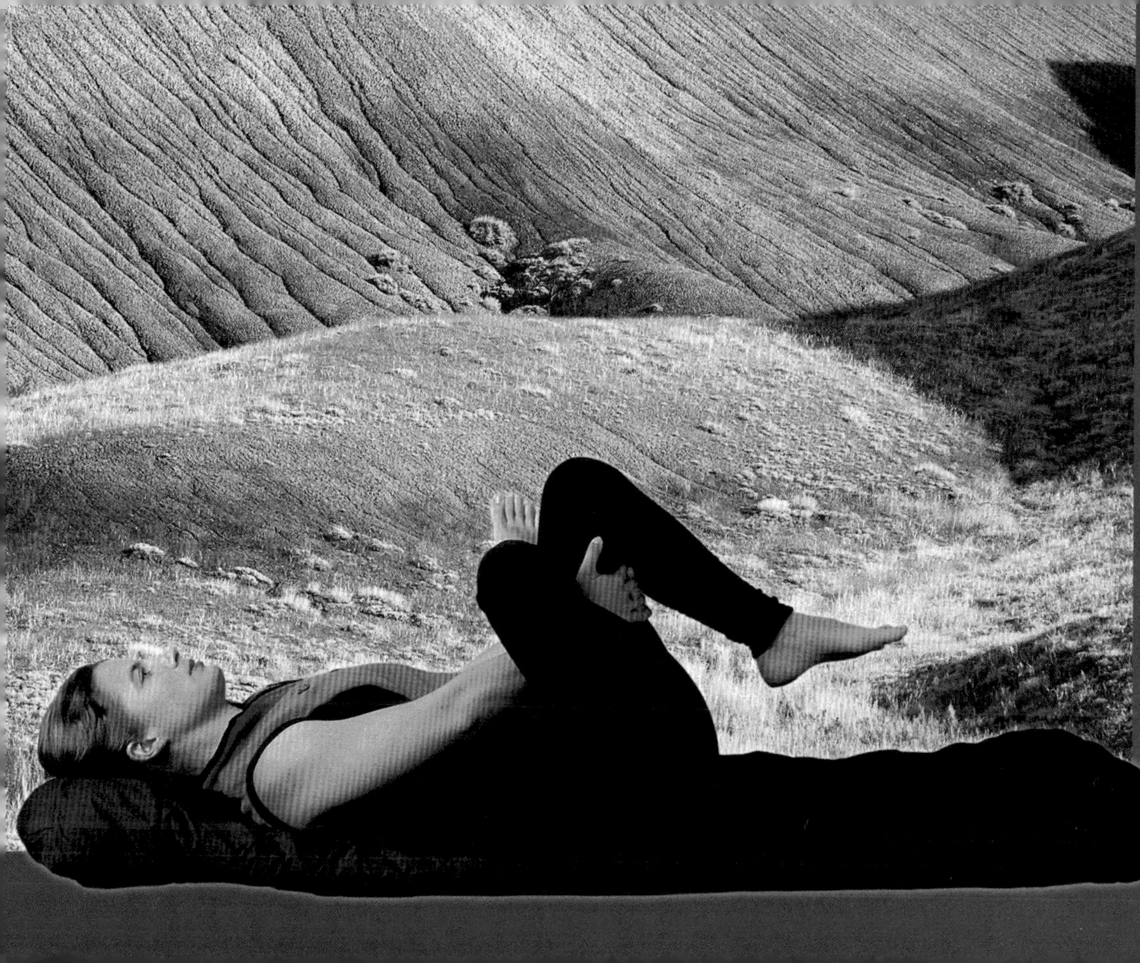

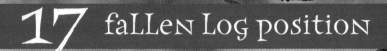

17 faLLen Log position

1 From Switchback Position, bring legs together and pull knees toward chest. Stretch arms out to either side at shoulder height, with palms facing down for stability. Rotate knees to one side and head toward the other.

2 Press knees toward ground, keeping shoulder blades flat against earth.

3 Use smooth, deep breathing to release tension in lower spine.

4 Repeat with opposite side.

yoga tip Bunch up a sleeping bag under your knees for support.

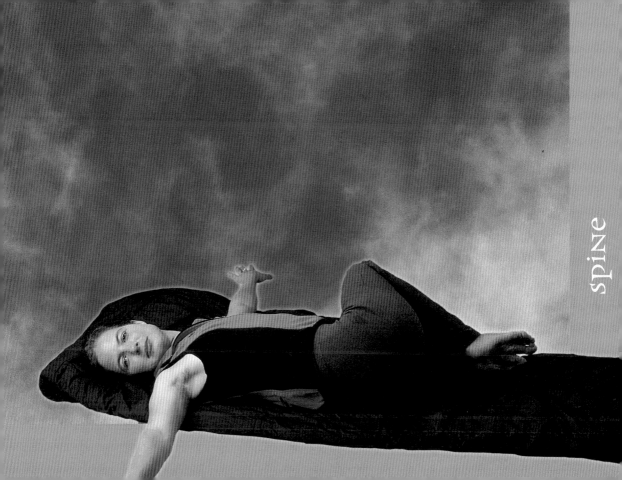

spine

18 many miLes position

1. Lie flat on belly. Bend one leg at knee. Reach back with hand to hold ankle and bring it alongside hip.

2. Press downward with pelvis and extend outward through knee.

3. Allow each breath to lengthen quadriceps muscle.

4. Repeat with opposite side.

sLeepinG baG tip Between trips, store your sleeping bag uncompressed to help preserve its loft.

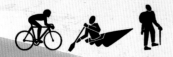

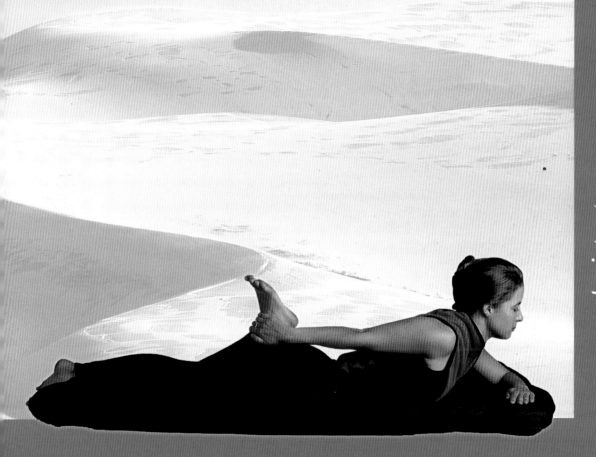

19 HIBERNATION POSITION

1 From Many Miles Position, draw both knees up and under chest, resting pelvis on heels and forehead on ground in front of you.

2 Stretch arms back toward feet, palms turned upward, and draw shoulder blades away from each other.

3 Relax your spine, softening any muscular tension and slowing down your body processes by focusing on your breathing.

yoga tip Rest your head on a sleeping bag or place one end of the bag behind your knees and under your thighs for additional support.

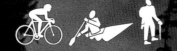

spine

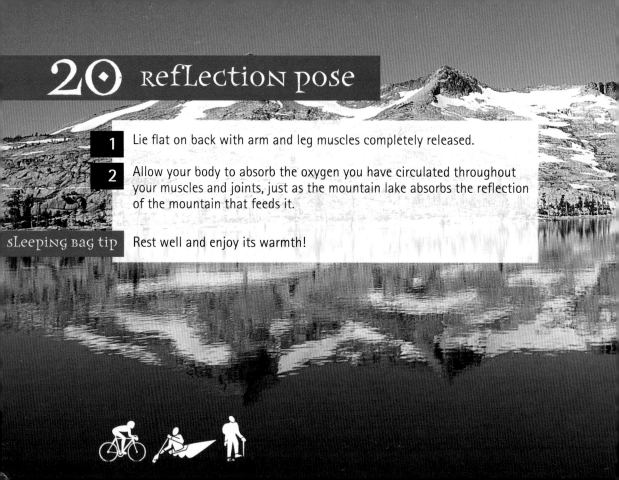

20 ◆ reflection pose

1 Lie flat on back with arm and leg muscles completely released.

2 Allow your body to absorb the oxygen you have circulated throughout your muscles and joints, just as the mountain lake absorbs the reflection of the mountain that feeds it.

sleeping bag tip Rest well and enjoy its warmth!

Rest

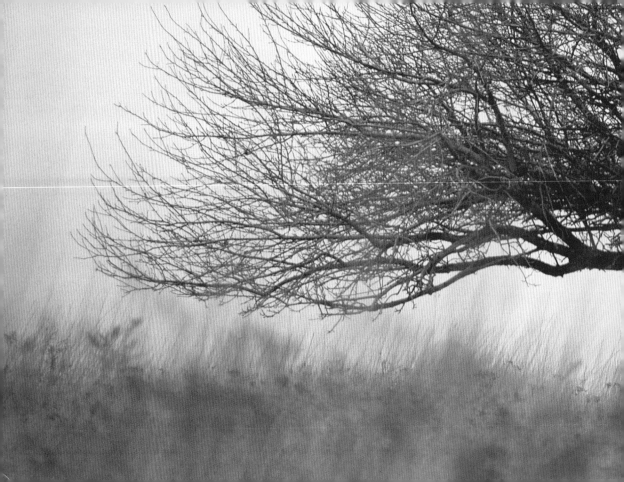

As you take that inevitable break between miles, practice the following Strengthening Series to rejuvenate your body. Doing this will actually release tension in overworked muscles, realign your spine, and prepare your muscles for further use. Over time, it will also strengthen the core body muscles you need to perform sports efficiently.

➤ The series demonstrates ten different positions. To complete a full series, begin with number 1 and move through all ten positions. Then, starting with number 6, work backward to number 1. You will end in the position in which you began, ready to repeat the series.

➤ As you practice the Strengthening Series, move smoothly from one position to the next on each breathing cycle: inhale in position, exhale as you change positions.

➤ Practice the complete series a couple of times in a row to keep your body warm and relaxed while increasing its strength.

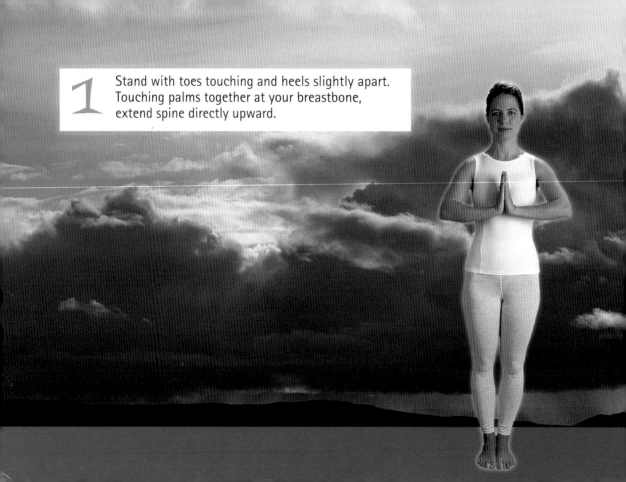

1 Stand with toes touching and heels slightly apart.
Touching palms together at your breastbone,
extend spine directly upward.

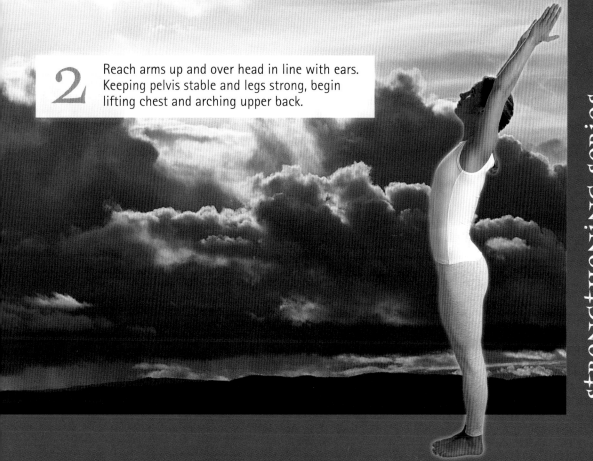

2 Reach arms up and over head in line with ears.
Keeping pelvis stable and legs strong, begin
lifting chest and arching upper back.

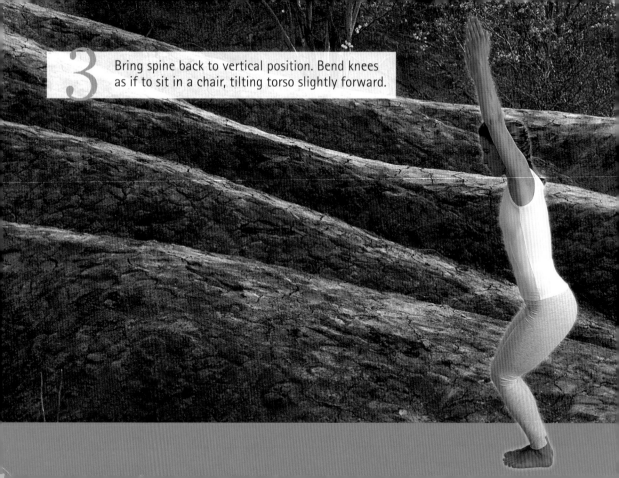

3 Bring spine back to vertical position. Bend knees as if to sit in a chair, tilting torso slightly forward.

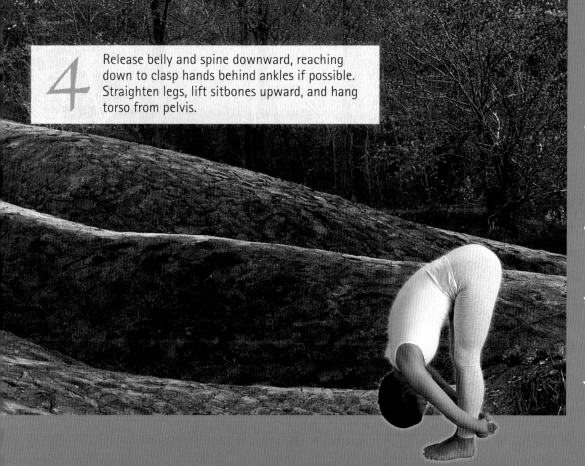

4 Release belly and spine downward, reaching down to clasp hands behind ankles if possible. Straighten legs, lift sitbones upward, and hang torso from pelvis.

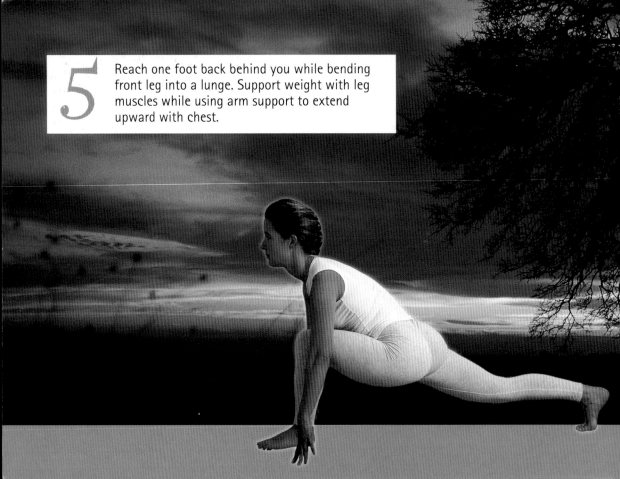

5 Reach one foot back behind you while bending front leg into a lunge. Support weight with leg muscles while using arm support to extend upward with chest.

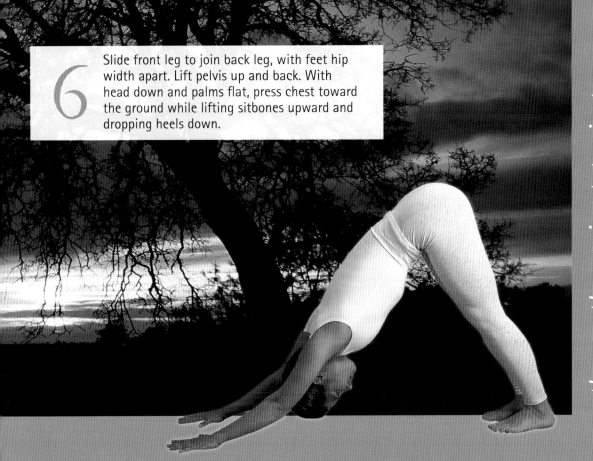

6 Slide front leg to join back leg, with feet hip width apart. Lift pelvis up and back. With head down and palms flat, press chest toward the ground while lifting sitbones upward and dropping heels down.

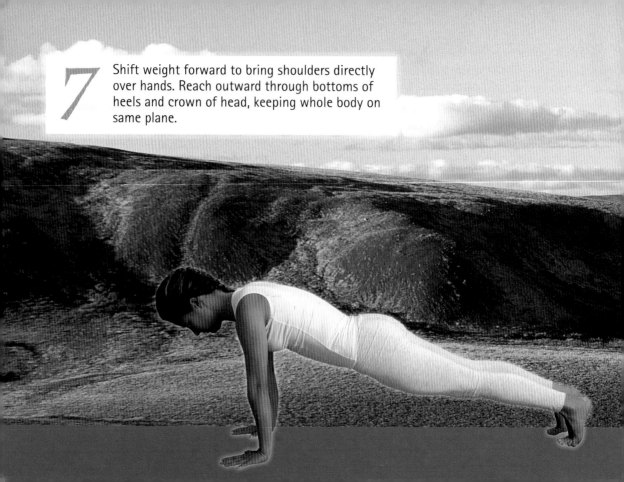

7 Shift weight forward to bring shoulders directly over hands. Reach outward through bottoms of heels and crown of head, keeping whole body on same plane.

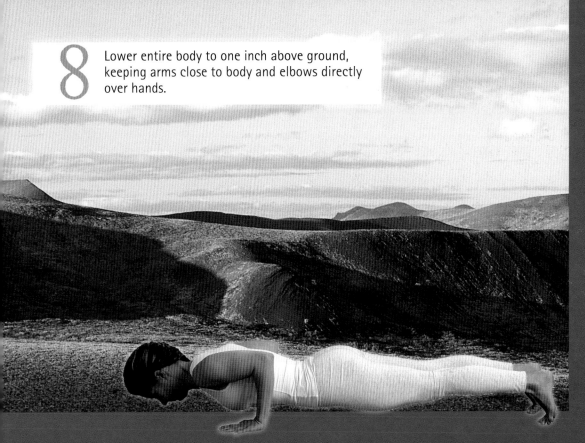

8 Lower entire body to one inch above ground, keeping arms close to body and elbows directly over hands.

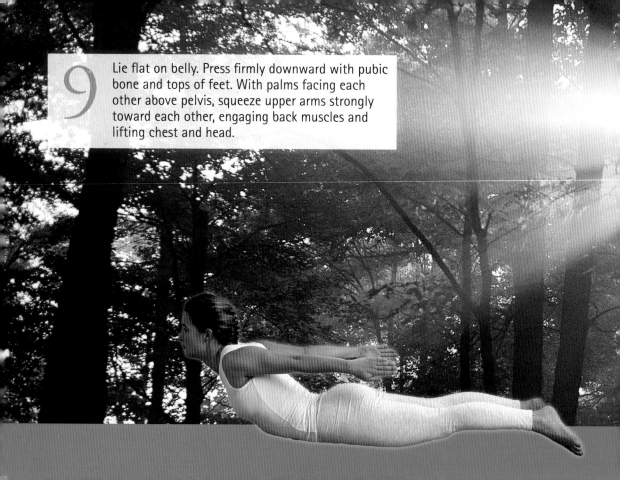

9 Lie flat on belly. Press firmly downward with pubic bone and tops of feet. With palms facing each other above pelvis, squeeze upper arms strongly toward each other, engaging back muscles and lifting chest and head.

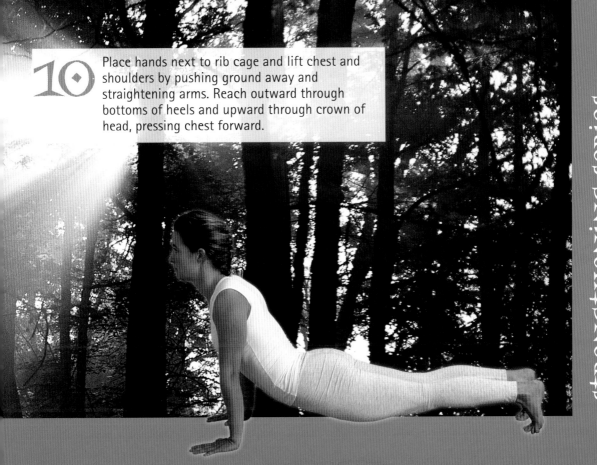

10 Place hands next to rib cage and lift chest and shoulders by pushing ground away and straightening arms. Reach outward through bottoms of heels and upward through crown of head, pressing chest forward.

► appendix

If you've practiced yoga before, some of the positions in *Sleeping Bag Yoga* will be familiar to you. For those who are interested, here is a list of the positions in this book with their corresponding Sanskrit and common Western names, when they exist.

	Sleeping Bag Yoga Name	Sanskrit Name	Common Western Name
1	Twilight	Virasana	Hero Pose
2	Moonlight	Virasana (variation)	Hero Pose (variation)
3	Ocean Swell		Cat and Cow Pose
4	Root ★	Adho Mukha Svanasana	
5	Mountain Pass	Adho Mukha Svanasana	Downward Facing Dog
6	New Growth	Urdhva Mukha Svanasana	Upward Facing Dog
7	Head Wind ★	Virabhadrasana I	Lunge Pose
8	Whirlpool	Marichyasana III	Twist
9	Sunrise	Parivitta Janu Sirasana	Revolved
10	Sunset	Janu Sirsasana	Head to Knee Pose
11	River Rock	Paschimottanasana	Seated Forward Bend
12	Crevasse		
13	Arches	Setu Banda	Bridge Pose
14	Valley Floor	Supta Baddha Konasana	Reclining Cobbler's Pose

★ Preparation for full Sanskrit position

15	Nurse Log		
16	Switchback		
17	Fallen Log ★	Jathara Parivartanasana	Revolved Belly Pose
18	Many Miles ★	Bhekasana	Frog Pose
19	Hibernation	Vajrasana	Child's Pose
20	Reflection	Savasana	Corpse Pose

▬ STRENGTHENING SERIES

	SANSKRIT NAME	COMMON WESTERN NAME
1	Tadasana	Mountain Pose
2	Tadasana (variation)	Mountain Pose (variation)
3	Utkatasana	Chair Pose
4	Uttanasana	Standing Forward Bend
5 ★	Virabhadrasana I	Warrior Pose
6	Adho Mukha Svanasana	Downward Facing Dog
7 ★	Chaturanga Dandasana	Plank Pose
8	Chaturanga Dandasana	Stick Pose
9 ★	Salabhasana	Locust Pose
10	Urdhva Mukha Svanasana	Upward Facing Dog